Barihely Bienvenido

Socio-familial factors associated with cannabis abuse

Barihely Bienvenido

Socio-familial factors associated with cannabis abuse

seen at the Morafeno Antsiranana psychiatric ward

ScienciaScripts

Imprint

Any brand names and product names mentioned in this book are subject to trademark, brand or patent protection and are trademarks or registered trademarks of their respective holders. The use of brand names, product names, common names, trade names, product descriptions etc. even without a particular marking in this work is in no way to be construed to mean that such names may be regarded as unrestricted in respect of trademark and brand protection legislation and could thus be used by anyone.

Cover image: www.ingimage.com

This book is a translation from the original published under ISBN 978-620-6-72027-0.

Publisher:
Sciencia Scripts
is a trademark of
Dodo Books Indian Ocean Ltd. and OmniScriptum S.R.L publishing group

120 High Road, East Finchley, London, N2 9ED, United Kingdom
Str. Armeneasca 28/1, office 1, Chisinau MD-2012, Republic of Moldova, Europe
Printed at: see last page
ISBN: 978-620-8-04213-4

DEDICATIONS AND THANKS

I dedicate this thesis :
TO ALMIGHTY GOD
"Not I, but the grace of God which is with me". 1 Corinthians 15:10
In memory of my grandfather BARIHELY Tombolahy and his wife SAKINA Georgette

"Ny hazo no vanon-kolakana, ny tany naniriany no tsara".
"I know you would have been proud of me if you were still in this world.

To my dear parents

"To whom I owe everything! For all the sacrifices they had to make to have a son

doctor".
"Your greatest desire has always been my success".

To my family

"Thank you for all your moral and financial support. Thank you to those who have always been there for me.

To all my class KINTANA

"My sincere thanks".

AT THE CATHOLIC UNIVERSITY CHAPLAINCY IN ANTSIRANANA

"Rise and shine". Isaiah 60:1

TO THE MAHAVAVY STUDENTS' ASSOCIATION

"Ambilobe tsy lany olo-manga".

To Doctor TONINA Roxane

"Thank you so much for all your help and advice during my thesis".

Doctor RAHARIVELO Adeline

- Professor of Higher Education and Research in Psychiatry at the Faculty of Medicine in Antananarivo.
- Vice-Dean of the Antananarivo Faculty of Medicine.

- Director of the Joseph Raseta Befelatanana Antananarivo University Hospital.

- Head of the Psychiatry Unit at Joseph Raseta Befelatanana Hospital Antananarivo.

Despite your heavy responsibilities and your many obligations, you have has done me the great honour of agreeing to supervise this thesis.

Thank you very much. Please accept our sincere gratitude.

Doctor RAKOTOARISOA Andriarimanana Hery Nirina

- Professor of Higher Education and Research in Otolaryngology and Cervicofacial Surgery at the Faculty of Medicine in Antsiranana.
- Head of Department of Otolaryngology and Cervicofacial Surgery at the Centre Hospitalier Universitaire de Place Kabary Antsiranana.
Doctor RANDRIAMBOLOLONA Domoina Malala Aurélia

- Associate Professor of Obstetrics and Gynaecology at the Faculty of Medicine of Antsiranana.

- Director of the Centre Hospitalier Universitaire de Place Kabary Antsiranana.
- Head of the Gynaecology and Obstetrics Department at the Tanambao I University Hospital in Antsiranana.

"You have done us the honour of sitting on the jury for our work. Please accept our sincere thanks and respect.

TO OUR THESIS RAPPORTEUR

Doctor ZANADAORY

- Lecturer in Higher Education and Research.

- Former Dean of the Antsiranana Faculty of Medicine.

- Head of Psychiatry at Morafeno Antsiranana.

"Who inspired us to write this thesis. You have guided us with sincerity and kindness throughout the realisation of this work. Please accept the expression of our deepest respect and admiration."

TO OUR MASTER AND DEAN OF THE FACULTY OF MEDICINE AT ANTSIRANANA

Madame le Docteur RAZAFINDRAZANANY Nelly Félicienne Our most respectful tributes.

TO ALL OUR MASTERS AND TEACHERS AT THE FACULTY OF MEDICINE IN ANTSIRANANA

AND HOSPITAL DOCTORS

Our respectful thanks in recognition of the teaching that you you have given us over so many years.

TO ALL THE ADMINISTRATIVE AND TECHNICAL STAFF OF THE FACULTY OF MEDICINE

D'ANTSIRANANA

Our sincere thanks.

TO ALL THE DOCTORS AND STAFF OF THE MORAFENO ANTSIRANANA PSYCHIATRY DEPARTMENT

Our warmest thanks.

TO ALL THOSE WHO, DIRECTLY OR INDIRECTLY, HAVE CONTRIBUTED TO THE PREPARATION OF THIS REPORT.

THESIS

Our sincere thanks.

CONTENTS

INTRODUCTION

Cannabis is a narcotic plant [1]. According to the WHO [2], it is one of the most widely used illicit substances worldwide. In 2013, 181.8 million people aged between 15 and 64 were estimated to have used cannabis at least once in their lives. Its use is a real public health problem, and seems to be of particular interest to young people.In Madagascar, there are as yet no exact figures reflecting the prevalence of cannabis use, despite the devastation caused by this product. But what is certain is that our country is certainly not spared from this problem. Youth is a time of experimentation, often including experimentation with drugs, especially as young people are a particularly vulnerable and impressionable group. The urban environment is a factor that encourages drug use. Cannabis use appears to be particularly widespread among the working population, compared with the unemployed and those with a low level of education [3]. The use of psychoactive substances by parents and peers and their approval of this use is the main social antecedent of adolescent cannabis use [4]. Other factors include disruption of family relationships, parental separation, psychiatric disorders in the family and deviant adolescents [5]. Psychological factors that precede cannabis use include difficulties at school, personality traits such as sensation or novelty seeking, aggression, impulsivity, low self-esteem and psychiatric disorders such as anxiety and depressive disorders, conduct disorders, hyperactivity and borderline personality [4].

A study carried out in the psychiatric department in Antsiranana in 2018 showed that cannabis is the most widely consumed illicit product, with a rate of 88.81% compared with other substances [6]. Abuse of this product poses serious problems for society and even for the State. This underlines the relevance of research into the socio-familial factors linked to cannabis abuse observed in patients admitted to the department.The aim of our work was to describe the socio-familial factors associated with cannabis abuse and to assess the types of substances associated with cannabis. Our work is divided into three parts: the first is devoted to background information, the second to methodology and results, and the last to discussion and suggestions.

PART ONE

BACKGROUND

I- HISTORY OF CANNABIS

I.1. History of man and cannabis

Cannabis is the most widely used illicit drug, with occasional, rarely abusive and stable use [7]. The plant originates from Central Asia and is also known as sativa indica or Indian hemp. Humans have used it since the dawn of time for its medicinal properties (antispasmodic, analgesic, etc.) and also for its euphoric properties, which were discovered in India in 2000 BC. It was introduced to Europe in the nineteenth century, brought by travellers from India to England, and since then its use has spread throughout the world, making it the most widely consumed illicit substance [8].

I.2. Legal background at Madagascar

In the past, the "Malagasy" ancestors used to smoke cannabis. King Andrianampoinimerina promulgated severe sentences formally prohibiting cannabis plantations in the territories of his kingdom. But, unbeknown to the King, the population consumed it all the same. In the 19th century, the Charters of the Traditional Collectivities of the Highlands condemned the use of cannabis [9]. Order no. 145/ CG of 23 May 1958 reiterated the ban on the cultivation and possession of cannabis. These texts were repealed by Order no. 60-073 of 28 July 1960, itself repealed by Law no. 97-039 of 4 November 1997 on the control of narcotics and psychotropic substances in Madagascar. The cultivation of opium poppies, coca bushes and cannabis plants is prohibited on national territory, and the owner, operator or occupier in any capacity whatsoever of land used for agricultural or other purposes is required to destroy any such plantations that may grow there [10].

II- NEUROBIOLOGY OF CANNABIS

II.1. Presentation of cannabis

It is a herbaceous plant belonging to the Cannabaceae family, with leaves cut into 5 to 7 lanceolate, toothed and fan-shaped characters. Its leaves bear hairs that secrete a resin rich in delta9 tetrahydrocannabinol (Δ^9 THC), which is the active ingredient responsible for the psychoactive effects of cannabis [11].

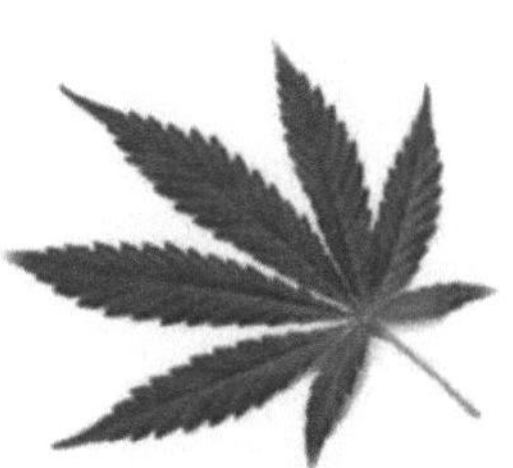

Figure 1: Cannabis leaf

II.2. Metabolism

Absorption of Δ9-THC is rapid because it is highly lipophilic. After inhalation or oral administration, around 15 to 50% of delta9 THC is absorbed very quickly and passes into the bloodstream. The dose-dependent maximum blood concentration is reached 7 to 10 minutes after inhalation. The absorbed delta9 THC is then metabolised in the liver microsomes to produce the following compounds [11-14]:

- 11-hydroxy-tetrahydrocannabinol is a psychoactive metabolite.
- 8 -beta hydroxy delta9 tetrahydrocannabinol is potentially psychoactive, but its contribution to the effects of cannabis is negligible due to its very low concentration and very rapid metabolism.

- 8 beta-11-dehydroxy-delta9-tetrahydrocannabbinol and 8-α-hydroxydelta9-tetrahydrocannabinol, which are not psychoactive.

THC is very quickly taken up by richly vascularised and fatty tissues such as the liver and brain, due to its lipophilic nature. A very slow process of elimination then takes place, with the consumption of a joint leaving THC in the brain for a week. It is eliminated by a number of different routes, and whatever the method of consumption, elimination is always very slow, mainly via the digestive tract, with 65-80% via the faecal route and 20-35% via the urinary tract.The rate of elimination varies from subject to subject, with an average half-life of 2 to 8 days, but this depends mainly on the dose ingested and the frequency of use.

II.3. Receptors cannabinoids

The discovery of THC as the active ingredient in cannabis in 1964 led to the discovery of cannabinoid receptors. There are two of these: CB1 receptors and CB2 receptors [15-17]:
- CB1 receptors were isolated from rat brain in 1988. They are mainly found centrally, especially in the cortex, hippocampus, amygdala and basal ganglia.
- CB2 receptors were isolated from myelocyte cells in 1993. They are few in number at central level, apart from the amygdala, but are mainly located in the immune system (lymphocytes, spleen, leukocytes, etc.), and appear to be

responsible for the immunomodulatory effects of cannabinoids. Stimulation of CB1 receptors activates numerous intracellular signalling pathways in the central nervous system and regulates the function of the and inhibiting certain calcium channels, thereby reducing neuronal excitability. This regulation of ion channels and the presynaptic location of CB1 receptors explain the inhibitory effects of cannabinoids on neurotransmitter release.

II.4. Ligands for endocannabinoid receptors

Three types of ligand are known today [18,19]:

- There are many natural exogenous ligands, represented by the cannabinoids identified in the cannabis sativa plant - over 60 according to the literature - but delta 9 THC is the most active, responsible for the psychoactive effects of cannabis.
- Endogenous ligands, derived from fatty acids, notably arachidonic acid. The main endocannabinoids are arachidonylethanolamide, known as anandamide, and 2-arachidonoyl-glycerol or 2-AG. Anandamide is present in various areas of the human brain (hippocampus, thalamus, cerebellum and striatum), while 2-AG has also been identified in the brain and spleen. Their release following post-synaptic stimulation then activates cannabinoid receptors.
- Finally, other synthetic ligands or cannabinoids.

II.5. Influence of cannabis on the dopaminergic system

In the particular case of the nucleus accumbens, the structure that contains the reward and addiction system, CB1 receptors are positioned on gabaergic neurons. Their stimulation therefore leads to a reduction in the secretion of the neurotransmitter GABA in the synaptic space. The large number of dopaminergic neurons present in this area, which are normally inhibited in the basal state by GABA (figure 1), will see their inhibition lifted, thereby increasing the secretion of dopamine, which may explain the behavioural and addictive effect of cannabis [19].

Figure 2. Diagrams showing effect of the stimulation of receptors presynaptic cannabinoids(CB1) by THC

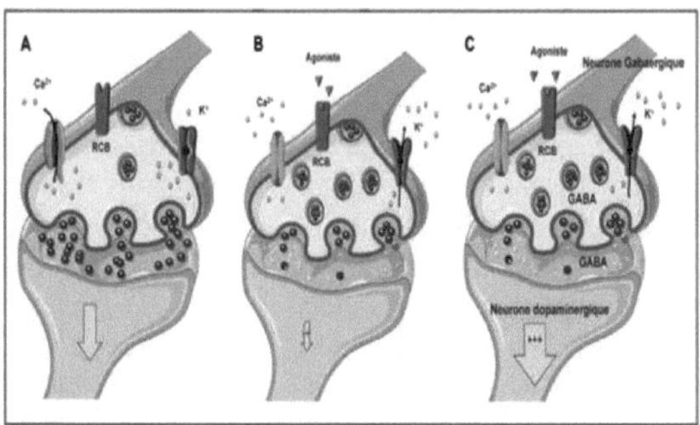

Source : Alvarez. JL, Pape. E,Stanislas GD,knapp. A. Synthetic cannabinoids: Pharmacological aspects.TOXAC 2014. [19]

A. Neuronal synapse in basal state

B. Neuronal synapse after stimulation of BCR1 resulting in a decrease in the release of neurotransmitters into the synaptic space, leading to a decrease in the general excitability of the neuron.

C. Special case of the nucleus accumbens. Stimulation of the RCB1 is at the origin of the decrease in GABA, leading to an increase in the release of dopamine.

II.6. Dosage

Until the late 1970s, cannabinoids were only detected in urine, as the other methods available were not very specific or sensitive. It was not until the development of more sensitive and more specific chromatographic methods that delta-9 HC and its metabolites could be identified and measured in other media [18].

Nowadays, it is possible to measure cannabis in various biological media (blood, urine, saliva, hair, sweat, etc.). The choice of medium(s) depends on the context and objective of the investigation [11,20] :

▪ Blood
It is the most appropriate biological fluid in the forensic context (road accidents) to confirm recent cannabis use.
Advantages: - Blood tests can differentiate between active ingredients and non-active metabolites.
- Estimate the time elapsed between the last drink and the blood test.

- Excellent sensitivity because the detection limit is 0.4ng/ml.
Techniques: gas chromatography with mass spectrometry detection or GC-MS is

currently the most reliable method. This method is validated and recommended by the French Society of Analytical Toxicology in the context of road safety.

In the blood, THC concentrations remain detectable generally 6 to 12 hours after inhalation for occasional users, and up to 24 to 48 hours for regular users.

▪ Urine

They are still the most appropriate sample for rapid detection of cannabis use, and are frequently used in road accidents, workplace drug testing, monitoring of drug addicts and anti-doping campaigns.

Technique: enzymatic technique or EMIT (enzymemultiplied immuassay technique), fluorescence immunopolarisation.

Advantage: rapid response in 5 to 10 minutes. Detection threshold: 50ng. After a single dose of THC, the urine test is generally positive as soon as the second hour and will remain so for 5 to 7 days, but sometimes up to 12 days. With repeated use, the detection time for THC and its metabolites in the urine increases to more than 2 months.

▪ Saliva

Excretion of cannabinoids from the bloodstream into the saliva is in fact very low or non-existent; it is more a matter of sequestration in the mouth and teeth during inhalation. Concentrations are very high in the minutes following inhalation, generally in excess of 1000 µg/l. This level declines very quickly, but remains detectable for 4 to 6 hours, or even 10 hours in the case of high inhalation doses.

▪ Sweat

It is a poor environment for investigation because it is exposed to external contamination.

▪ Hair

THC concentrations are of the order of a few nanograms per milligram of hair, requiring the use of high-performance chromatographic techniques.Advantages: can be used to establish chronicity and level of use, and to monitor abstinence, making it useful for forensic medicine, occupational medicine and anti-doping purposes.

III- EPIDEMIOLOGY

III.1. Overall view of drug use

In 2015, some 246 million people aged between 15 and 64 had used drugs in 2013, representing an increase of 3 million individuals compared with the previous year, but because of the increase in the world's population, drug use is thought to have remained stable. The interest in this subject seems obvious when we consider that more than one drug user in ten is a problem drug user, i.e. has problems related to drug use, both somatic and psychological [21]. In 2010, the prevalence of problem drug users was estimated at between 10 and 13% [22]. In 2014, the number of drug users rose to 250 million among people aged 15-64, and around 207400 deaths, or 43.5 deaths per million inhabitants, are thought to be linked to drug use [23].

Cannabis is still by far the most widely used drug in the world. according to the UNODC in its 2004 report [24].

III.2. Consumption of cannabis

III.2.1. Population

III.2.1.1. At worldwide

Cannabis is not only the most widely used illicit substance in the world, it is also the leading psychoactive substance consumed during adolescence. In 2011, it was estimated that around 42% of 17-year-olds would have smoked cannabis at least once in their lives, with a high prevalence among males [25].

According to the European report on drugs in 2017, around 17.1 million young Europeans aged between 15 and 34 have smoked cannabis in the past year, with a predominance of males, and the average age of initiation was 16 [26]. In 2004, the UNODC estimated that 146.2 million people, or 3.7% of the population aged between 15 and 65, had used cannabis at least once in their lives [24]. This figure has tended to increase over the years: in 2009, according to the UNODC, there were around 190 million cannabis users in the world [27], and 119-224 million cannabis users in 2010 [22].

III.2.1.2. At Africa

In 2005, Africa was considered to be one of the world's biggest users of cannabis, with a prevalence rate of 7.7%, or 38,20,000 of the population aged between 15 and 64, and a rate well above 3.8% of global users [28]. In 2010, the annual prevalence rate of drug use was estimated at between 5.2 and 13.5% of the population aged 15 to 64 [22].

III.2.1.3. A Madagascar

A study was carried out in the psychiatric department of the CHU Joseph Raseta Befelatanana during 2016, with a view to identifying the sociodemographic and clinical factors associated with cannabis use. This study showed that among the 201 patients who presented with psychotic disorders, 40% had already used cannabis at least once in their lives [29]. In 2013, 13.75% of the 600 secondary school students had already used cannabis in the course of their lives, according to a study conducted in 6 secondary schools in the city of Antananarivo to determine the epidemiological profile of drug use among secondary school students [30].

III.2.2. Population psychiatric

The association of "psychiatric disorder" and "cannabis use" is more frequent than in the general population [31]. It is even said that people suffering from psychiatric disorders use approximately twice as much psychoactive substances as the general population. According to a study by Thomas et al, 47% of people with schizophrenia have a history of substance abuse, compared with 13.5% to 17% of the general population [32,33]. This association is like a double-edged sword, because if the aim of taking this product was to relieve the symptoms [34], According to some studies, it is a factor that aggravates the disease and could even worsen the prognosis. The average prevalence of cannabis use in these patients is 40% [35].

IV- CONSUMPTION

IV.1. Start of consumption

The socio-educational workers agree that they observe the start of consumption at around age 15. The circumstances in which young people start using are also varied: either at a party, or with older friends, or their older brother or a friend's older brother, or with friends or neighbourhood friends, or with their older boyfriend in the case of young women. The motivations for first use are mainly festive and experimental, linked to groups and peers. On the other hand, one common feature characterises the start of everyone's consumption: the first joints are offered by others, never bought by new users [36].

IV.2. Frequency and quantity of consumption

Akré et al reported in a study that 16 daily users smoked several joints a day. Some started smoking in the morning, others at lunchtime, and others smoked only in the evening when they left school or work and went to bed. Their consumption increases at weekends and during holidays - in other words, during times when they socialise with their peers [36].

IV.3. Mode taken

There are various ways of consuming cannabis [37] :
- Inhalation: either by inhaling smoke such as joints and pipes, or by inhaling hemp vapours using a vaporiser.
- Oral, in pill and oil form.

- Sublingual route in spray form.

- Applied to the skin as a cream.

V- **VULNERABILITY FACTORS**

No smoker is born a smoker. We must always look for the factors that trigger this tendency. Certain so-called vulnerability factors have been identified on the basis of the results of studies, and are grouped into 2 groups: individual and environmental factors [38-40] :

V.1. **Individual risk factors**

The following table (Table I) summarises the various individual factors that could be responsible for taking the drugs.

Table I. Individual risk factors (personality traits, temperament, behaviour)

Traits de personnalité	Tempérament	Comportement
-Faible estime de soi	-Faible évitement du danger	-Tendance agressive
-Timidité	-Faible niveau de sociabilité -	
-Autodépréciation	Niveau élevé de recherche de nouveautés	-Turbulent
-Réactions émotionnelles excessives		- Impulsivité
-Difficultés à faire face à certains évènements	-Retour lent à l'équilibre après un stress	
-Difficultés à avoir des relations stables		
-Difficultés à résoudre les problèmes interpersonnels		
-Psychotasisme (attitude antisociale, haut degré d'hostilité, rejets des normes culturelles)		

In addition to personality traits, temperament and behaviour, there are other factors :

▪ Life events
Life events such as bereavement, break-ups, mistreatment, sexual abuse, homelessness and serious somatic illnesses play an important role in the onset of substance abuse.

▪ Psychiatric comorbidities
According to studies in this field, the existence of a psychiatric pathology increases the risk of developing abuse of or dependence on a psychoactive substance by a factor of 2. In most cases, these disorders precede drug use, and may include mood disorders (depression, bipolar disorder), anxiety disorders (phobia, generalised anxiety disorder, post-traumatic stress disorder), eating disorders, conduct disorders or attention deficit hyperactivity disorder.

V.2. Risk factors

V.2.1. Family factors

Intra-familial functioning, family ties and parental education style (neglectful, rejecting, permissive) are thought to play a major role in the genesis of illicit substance use in children. In addition, the use of illicit substances by one of the parents, especially the mother, family tolerance for the use of substances and the breaking of family rules increase the likelihood of children and adolescents using illicit substances.

V.2.2. Factors social

- Socio-cultural environment

Disruption, exclusion from school and a lack of educational support leave children and teenagers to fend for themselves without any reference points or protective barriers, making them vulnerable to outside temptations, especially from friends.The loss of social references such as unemployment, poverty, precariousness, lack of moral values and marginalisation are strongly correlated with the use of psychoactive substances.

- Our friends

From adolescence onwards, the influence of parents on substance use diminishes, while that of peers increases considerably. In fact, experimentation with substances in adolescence depends to a large extent on the friends who use them. In addition, the initiation of substance use is much more likely to be influenced by a close friend than by a stranger.

VI- CANNABIS AND PSYCHIATRIC DISORDERS

Cannabis is responsible for clinical manifestations such as cannabis-induced drunkenness, psychotic disorders, amotivational syndrome, anxiety disorders, cognitive disorders, depressive disorders and suicide.

VI.1. Drunkenness cannabique

This is a genuine psychotic experience, the manifestations of which are according to the dose ingested, as shown in table 2 [41].

Table II. Clinical presentation as a function of dose

A faible dose < 50µg/kg	Forte dose > 200µg/kg
Sentiment d'euphorie	Etats de dépersonnalisation
Modifications des perceptions du temps	Déréalisation
Modification de la perception de l'espace et de la personnalité	Distorsion
	Illusions visuelles et auditives
	Etats confuso-oniriques

VI.2. psychotic disorder

Cannabis can give rise to psychotic disorders which are characterised by the suddenness of their onset, the association with self- and/or heteroaggressive behavioural disorders, auditory and also visual psychosensory manifestations, a delusional syndrome with a polymorphic theme, psychomotor disinhibition and rapid regression under rapid neuroleptic treatment, with criticism of the episode [41].
The question that arises is the role of cannabis in the genesis or precipitating factor in the onset of a psychotic disorder in a subject with premorbid risk factors. To avoid any confusion, a distinction should be made between two types of psychotic disorder induced by cannabis: toxic psychosis and functional psychosis [42].

➤ Functional psychosis: characterised by its longer duration (two weeks), the clinical features include a syndrome of depersonalisation, elements of hypomania, disorganised thinking and sometimes both visual and auditory hallucinations. It occurs in smokers with vulnerability factors such as schizothymic personality traits.
➤ Toxic psychosis lasts a few days and is characterised by somatic symptoms such as confusion and disorientation. It generally occurs in inexperienced users who are not psychotic.

Cannabis use in patients suffering from schizophrenia aggravates delusional, hallucinatory and disorganised symptoms. It also worsens the long-term course of the disease, with more frequent hospitalisations, poor compliance with treatment and social exclusion [43].

VI.3. Amotivational syndrome

The ability of cannabis to induce amotivational syndromes was described by Ball in 1894. This disorder combines a lack of activity, emotional indifference and physical and intellectual asthenia, with poverty and slowing down. This syndrome is associated with long-term, continuous drug use, and regresses after a few weeks to a few months of abstinence [43].

VI.4. Anxiety disorders

These are probably the most frequent complications and are often the reason for stopping intoxication, but they reappear when the drug is taken again. A distinction is made between [44]:

➤ A panic attack or "bad trip" is a sudden onset of paroxysmal anxiety lasting from a few minutes to a few hours.
➤ Depersonalisation syndrome is a long-lasting anxiety disorder, lasting from a few months to a year. It is characterised by a feeling of strangeness with an experience of weirdness. There are no delusional or hallucinatory symptoms, and no disturbance of the train of thought.

VI.5. Cognitive disorders

VI.5.1. Cognitive impairment induced by a single dose in humans

Within 6 hours of its consumption, cannabis induces attention and memory problems, particularly working memory. We There is also a slowing of reaction time and impairment of executive functions, particularly planning and decision-making [18].

VI.5.2. Cognitive disorders induced by chronic consumption in men

Regular cannabis use is the cause of lasting cognitive impairment, which depends on the amount of cannabis consumed, the length of exposure and how early the first dose is taken. These disorders are :

➤ Attention and memory problems: according to numerous studies, chronic cannabis use (at least once a week for at least three years) is frequently associated with cognitive problems, in particular attention, working memory, prospective memory and episodic memory, with impaired encoding, storage and recall of information, as well as problems processing the information needed for decision-making [18].
➤ Impairment of executive functions: regular cannabis use is associated with impairment of executive functions such as planning, adaptive skills, ability to establish properties, mental flexibility, problem solving and creative ability [18].

VI.6. Depressive disorder and suicide

According to numerous studies, cannabis abuse increases the risk of depression fivefold [45]. It also significantly increases the risk of suicide attempts when there is an associated psychiatric disorder [18].

VII- SOMATIC COMPLICATIONS OF CANNABIS

Compared with the physical health of the general population, cannabis users are more exposed to various somatic problems, the consequences of which vary according to the duration of exposure, as shown in Table III [44].

Table III. Somatic complications of cannabis

Consommation aigue	Consommation chronique
- Cardiovasculaire :	-Cardiovasculaire :
Tachycardie, palpitation,	infarctus de myocarde, artérite.
Hypertension artérielle, fibrillation auriculaire,	
Bloc auriculoventriculaire.	
-Broncho-pulmonaire :	-Broncho-pulmonaire :
bronchodilalation se manifestant par	bronchite chronique (toux chronique,
des toux grasses, wheezing.	expectoration et râles bronchiques).
-Autres :	-Risque de cancer surtout :
mydriase, sècheresse buccale,	cancer broncho-pulmonaire,
hyperémie conjonctivale.	voies aériennes supérieures, langue.

PART TWO
METHODS AND RESULTS

I- METHODS

I.1. the study

The study was conducted at the Morafeno Antsiranana Psychiatry Department. It is located on the road to the University of Antsiranana, to the east of the "Y" junction.The department is staffed by two doctors, the head of whom is a specialist in neuropsychiatry, and the other a specialist in psychiatry. The medical team includes a senior mental health nurse, two mental health nurses and two support staff.This department receives and treats patients with neuropsychiatric disorders. Patient care is ensured by perfect coordination between the above-mentioned doctors and the nurses. Morafeno's psychiatric ward has two doctors' offices, a department head's office, a treatment room, eleven inpatient wards, four isolation rooms and two toilets.

I.2. Type of study

This was a retrospective, descriptive, cross-sectional, single-centre study.

I.3. Period of study

This study was carried out over a three-year period from 1er January 2017 to 31 December 2019.

I.4. Duration of the study

This project took 16 months to complete.

I.5. Population study

The study population consisted of all patients with cannabism hospitalised on the psychiatric ward during the study period.

I.6. Inclusion criteria

-   All hospitalised patients who had used cannabis at the study site during the study period were included in this study, with complete and well-filled records.

I.7. Non inclusion criteria

-   non-cannabolic patients hospitalised for other reasons were non included.

I.8. Exclusion criteria

- Patients hospitalised for cannabis use with incomplete or incorrectly completed records were excluded.

I.9. Sample size

Sampling was exhaustive.

I.10. The variables studied

The variables studied were as follows:

- Socio-familial data: age, gender, profession, level of education, marital status of patient and parents, siblings, criminal record, parenthood, guardian's drug habits, group attended, cannabis education campaign.
- Data on cannabis: age of onset, method of use, reason for use, length of use, substances associated with cannabis.
- Clinical data: reason for admission, clinical manifestations, psychiatric history.

I.11. Method of collecting data

The study materials consisted of :

- Clinical records of patients who have consumed cannabis which was found in their toxic history
- In-patient register
- Patient discharge register

I.12. Analysis of data

The data was collected using a pre-established survey form (see appendix) and processed using Microsoft ® Office Excel 2016 software.

I.13. Determining the sample size

As the sampling was exhaustive, we did not calculate the sample size, but set a minimum number of 30 patients to be included.

I.14. Limits of the study

This study was limited to patients admitted to the psychiatric department of Morafeno Antsiranana. It does not reflect all the socio-familial factors of the general population of Antsiranana. Similarly, patient recruitment was based solely on medical observation and not on biological evidence.

I.15. Ethical considerations

We had the agreement and authorisation of the Centre's line managers Place

Kabary University Hospital, before collecting patient data.Respect for confidentiality was paramount, and the data was kept confidential. kept on paper in a locked place inaccessible to other people.Medical confidentiality was preserved insofar as the patients' names were not included in the study.

II- RESULTS

II-1-Global data

Table IV. Breakdown of patients admitted to the department.

	Number of employees (n)	Percentage (%)
Inpatients	551	100
Cannabinoid patients	137	24,9
Selected patients	88	16

We identified 551 patients hospitalised on the psychiatric ward during the study period, 88 of whom were included.

II-2- Socio-family data II-2-1- Age
II-2-1-1- Average age

The mean age of our patients was 24.43 years, with a standard deviation of 5.02. The youngest patient was 14 and the oldest 45.

II-2-1-2- Breakdown by age group :

Table V. Breakdown of patients by age group

Age group (years)	Number of employees (n)	Percentage (%)
≤15	2	2,3
16-20	28	31,9
21-25	25	28,4
26-30	22	25
31-35	7	7,9
36-40	1	1,1
41-45	3	3,4
Total	88	100

The 16-20 age group was the most represented, at 31.9%.

II-2-2-Distribution according to gender

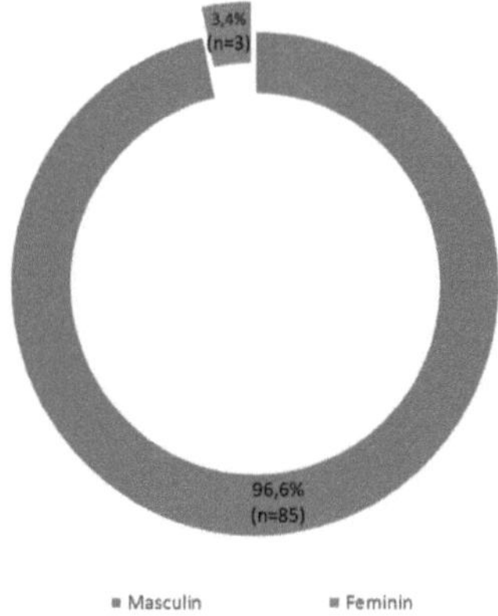

Figure 3: Distribution of patients by gender.

The figure shows that 96.6% of consumers are male.

II-2-3- Breakdown by occupation

II-2-3-1-By profession of consumers

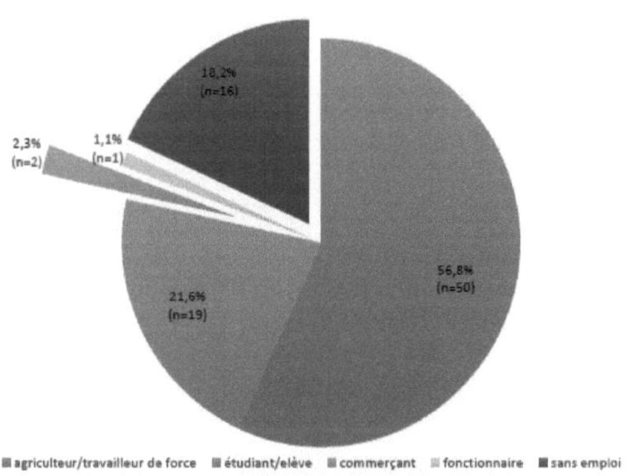

Figure 4: Breakdown of consumers by profession.
Farmers and forced labourers made up 56.8% of our samples.

II-2-3-2- According to the occupation of the parents or guardians of consumers

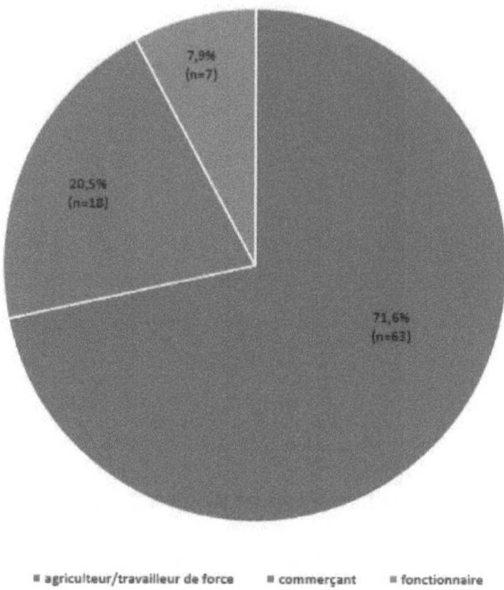

Figure 5: Breakdown by occupation of consumers' parents or guardians.
Among the consumers selected in our study, 71.6% of their parents had been farmers or forced labourers.

II-2-4-Distribution by level of study

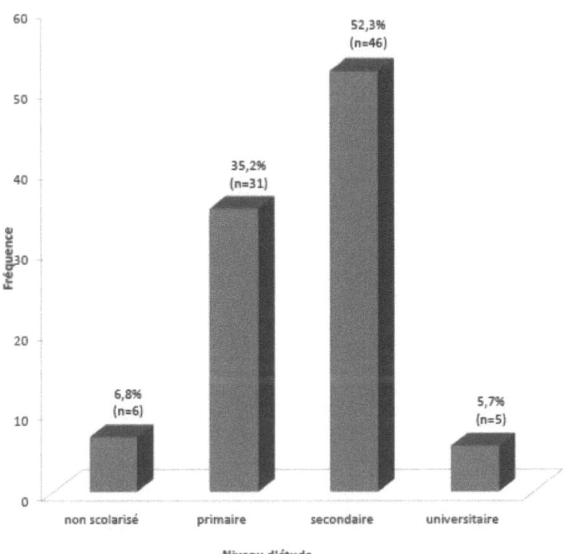

Figure 6. Distribution of patients by level of study.

Forty-six (46) or 52.3% of cannabis users had completed secondary education.

II-2-5- Breakdown by marital status

II-2-5-1-By marital status of patients

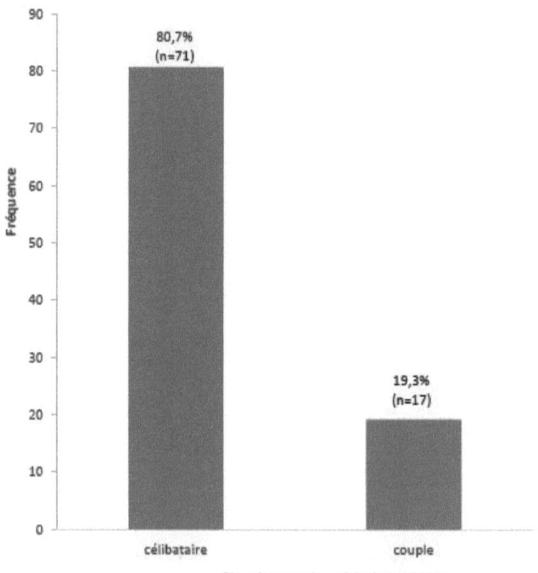

Figure 7.Breakdown of patients by marital status.
Cannabinoid patients were single in 80.7% of our samples.

II-2-5-2-According to the marital status of consumers' parents or guardians

Of the 88 cannabis-using patients, 63.6% (n=56) lived in single-parent families and 36.4% (n=32) lived in two-parent families.

II-2-6-Distribution according to parenthood

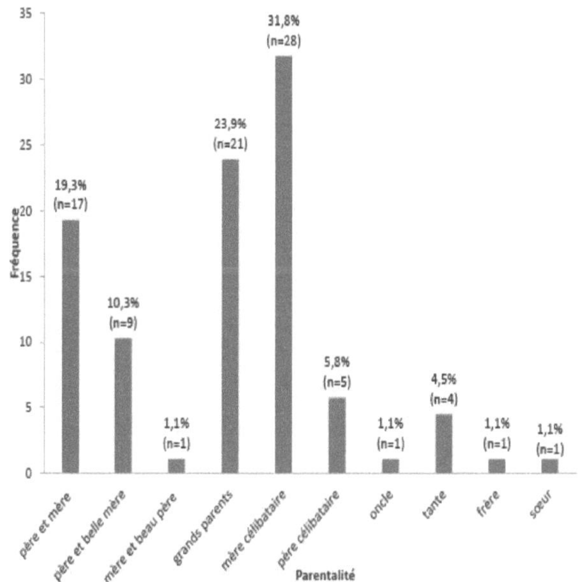

Figure 8: Distribution of patients according to parenthood.
Of the 88 patients, 31.8% had single mothers.

II-2-7-Distribution according to siblings II-2-7-1-Rank in siblings

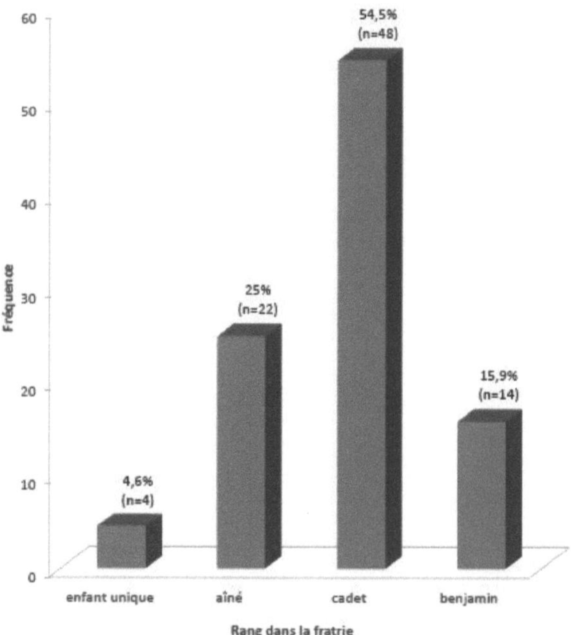

Figure 9: Distribution of patients according to sibling rank.
Cadets were the hardest hit, with a rate of 54.5%.

II-2-8- Breakdown by criminal record

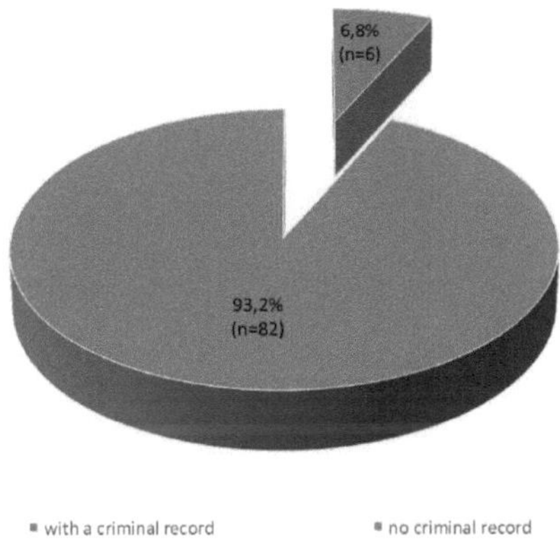

Figure 10: Breakdown of patients by criminal record.
Eighty-two (82), or 93.2% of the users, had no medical or legal history.

II-2-9- Toxic habits of parents or guardians

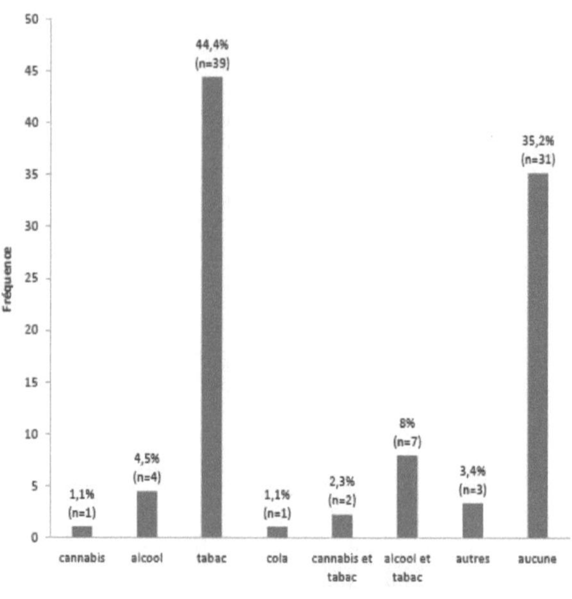

Figure 11: Distribution of parents' toxic habits

Thirty-nine (39) or 44.4% of the parents of the consumers were smokers.

II-2-10- Breakdown by group frequented and mode of consumption II-2-10-1- Group frequented

Table VI. Breakdown of patients by group attended.

Group attended	Number of employees (n)	Percentage (%)
Consumer	88	100
Non-consumer	00	00
Total	88	100

All the users, i.e. 100%, have been with consumers.

II-2-10-2-Mode of consumption

Table VII. Breakdown of patients by mode of consumption.

	Number of employees (n)	Percentage (%)
Smokes alone	6	6,8
Group smoking	82	93,2
Total	88	100

Eighty-two (82) or 93.2% of users smoked in groups.

II-2-11-Distribution according to the training and awareness campaign on cannabis

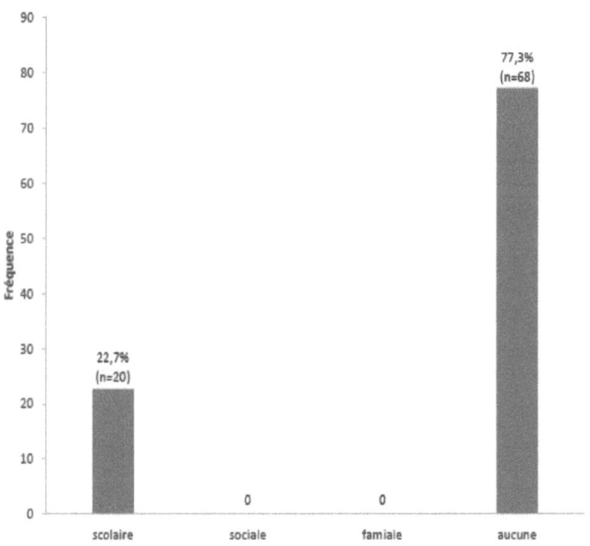

Figure 12.Breakdown of patients by cannabis education and awareness campaign.

The majority of users (77.3%) have not had any education about cannabis.

II-3- Data on cannabis

II-3-1-Age of first use at cannabis

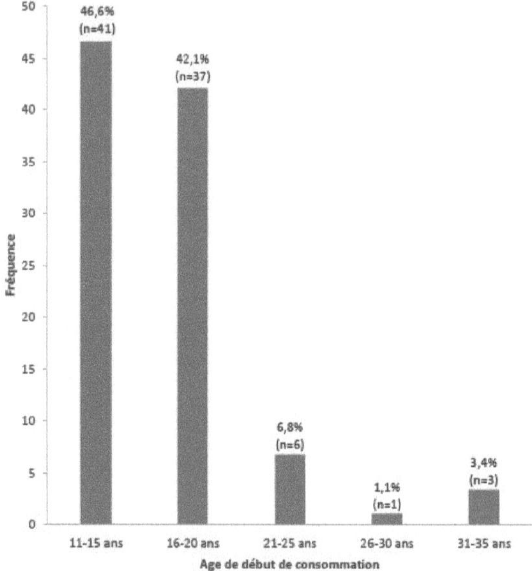

Figure 13: Distribution of patients by age of cannabis initiation.

The age at which cannabis use began varied between 11 and 15 years in 46.6% of cases.

II-3-2- Breakdown by type of taken

Forty-eight (88) or 100% of the users took cannabis by inhalation, all of them in the form of smoke.

II-3-3- Breakdown by frequency of use of cannabis

Table VIII. Distribution of patients according to frequency of cannabis use.

Frequency	Number of employees (n)	Percentage (%)
Occasional	04	4,5
Regular	84	95,5
Total	88	100

The majority (95.5%) were regular users who consumed according to a specific pattern (daily or weekly).

II-3-4-Distribution according to frequency of cannabis use for regular users

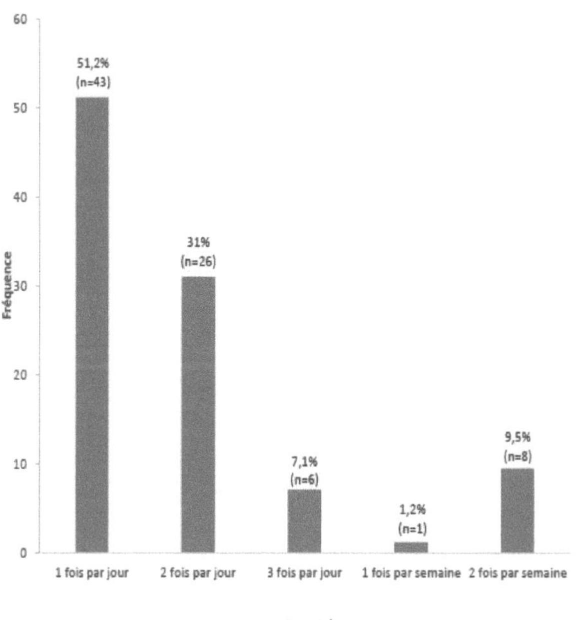

Figure 14: Breakdown of patients by frequency of cannabis use for regular cannabis use Figure 14

Of the 84 patients who used cannabis regularly, 43 (51.2%) used it once a day.

Of the regular users, 93.2% had consumed only one joint per session.

II-3-5- Breakdown by reason for consumption

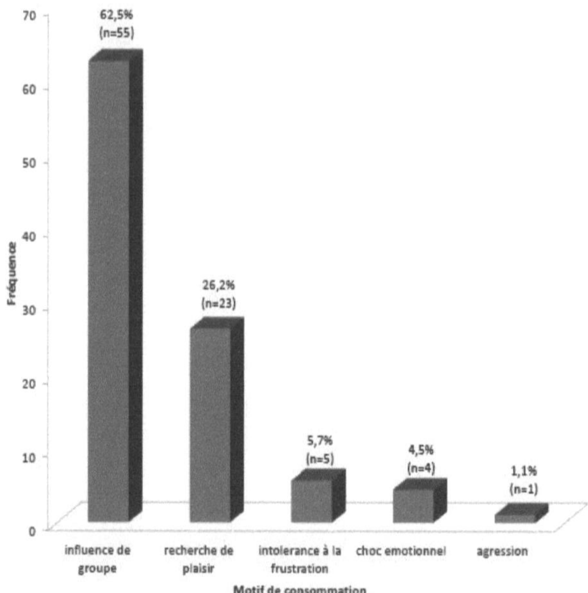

Figure 15: Breakdown of patients by reason for use.

The predominant reason for consumption was group influence at a rate of 62.5%.

II-3-6- Breakdown by age of consumption

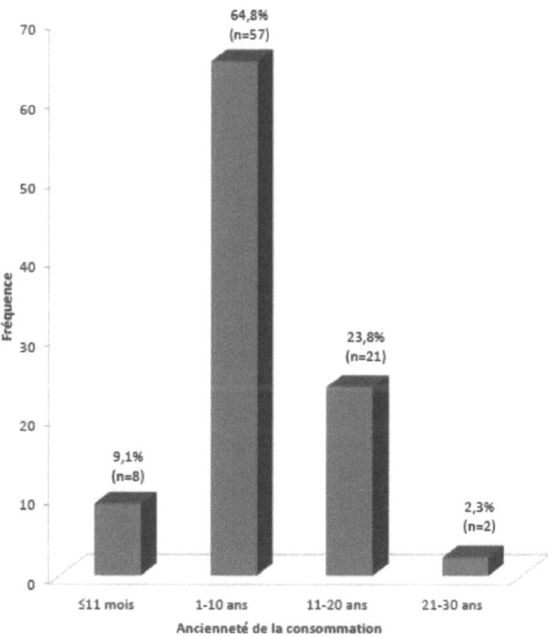

Figure 16: Breakdown of patients according to how long they have been using the drug

The average duration of use was 7.68 years, with a standard deviation of 4.35. The majority of users (64.8% of our samples) had been using cannabis for 1-10 years.

II-3-7-Associated substances

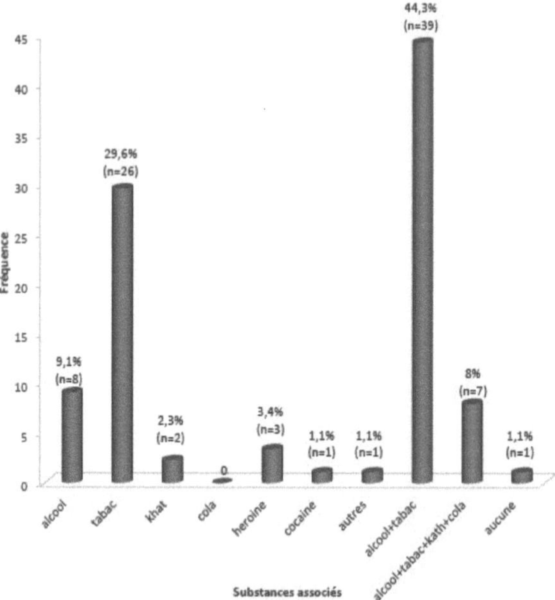

Figure 17: Distribution of patients according to substances associated with cannabis.

Thirty-nine (39) or 44.3% of our patients associated it with other psychoactive substances such as alcohol and tobacco.

II-4-Clinical data

II-4-1-Rationale for admission

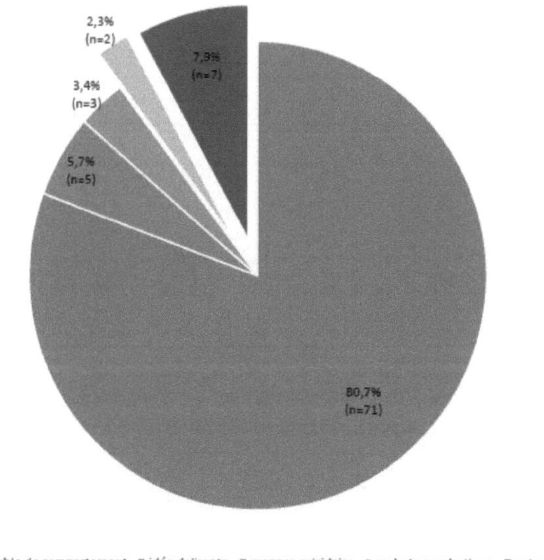

Figure 18. Breakdown of patients by reason for admission.
The majority of our patients (80.7%) were admitted for behavioural problems.

II-4-2- Distribution according to clinical symptoms

Among the 88 cannabis-using patients, psychotic symptoms were observed in 77.3% (n=68) of our samples, mood disorders in 15.9% (n=14) and social conduct disorders in 6.8% (n=6).

II-4-2-1-Psychotic symptoms

II-4-2-1-1-Delirium
The main themes presented by these psychotic patients were :
- Persecution (5 patients)

- Religious mysticism (12 patients)

- The idea of greatness (21 patients)

- Polymorphic (30 patients)

II-4-2-1-2- Hallucination

Table IX. Breakdown of patients by type of hallucination

Types of hallucinationNumber (n)	Percentage (%)	
Hearing 33	51,6	
Visual 27	42,2	
Psychic 3	4,7	
Cenesthesia 1	1,6	
Olfactory 0	0	
Total 64	100	
In our study, 64 psychotic patients	(94.1%) presented	from

hallucinations.

The table summarises the different types of hallucinations, with auditory hallucinations predominating at 51.6%.

II-4-2-1-3-Deficit signs

Three of our psychotic patients (4.4%) presented with deficits.

II-4-3- Psychiatric history

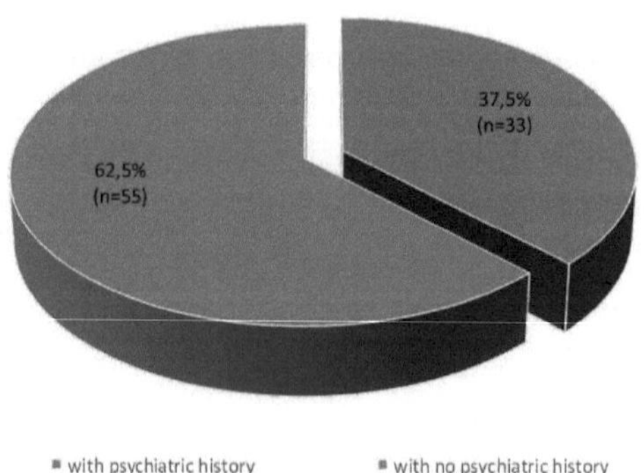

Figure 19: Distribution of patients according to psychiatric history.
Fifty-five (55) or 62.5% of the users had no psychiatric history.

PART THREE
DISCUSSION AND SUGGESTIONS

I- DISCUSSION

I-1-Global data

Among patients admitted to hospital during our study period, 16% of patients were included.A study carried out in Toulouse by Jouanjus, on the identification of serious complications associated with the use of psychoactive substances, estimated that 19.1% of patients suffered from cannabism over a 2-year study period [46].In a 3-year retrospective study conducted by Geus et al in Belgium to determine the psychotic disorder associated with cannabis use, the prevalence of cannabis-using patients was 37.5% [47].Our study differs from other studies in that it is based on patients who admitted to using cannabis during questioning and who were recorded in the files. Biological tests to determine THC levels are not available here, and the sample size does not represent the population of our town or the people admitted.

I-2-Family socio-data

I-2-1-Patient demographics

I-2-1-1-Age
In our study, the average age of patients was 24.43 years, with a minimum age of 14 and a maximum age of 45. The 16-20 age group was the most represented, with a proportion of 31.9%. In a study carried out in Saint Denis by Obradovic [48] as part of a consultation for young drug users, the average age of the patients was 21 years and 2 months, and the majority of these patients were between 14 and 25 years old, the youngest being 10 years old and the oldest 59 years old. Another study carried out in Morocco by Radia T [49], in her thesis entitled psychotic disorder and cannabis use, found an average age of 30 years. The youngest patient was 21 and the oldest 56, and the majority of these patients were aged between 25 and 30 (44%).Another study carried out in France by Guillem et al [50], looking at socio-demographic factors, found an average age of 27.5 years. The youngest patient was 15 and the oldest 51.According to the study conducted by Alson [29], in Antananarivo, the average age was 25.34 years, with the youngest being 15 years old and the oldest 56 years old; the majority of these patients were between 15 and 20 years old.
Our results are in line with those of previous studies. The young age is particularly a phase of physical and psychological pubertal transformation. This makes them all the more vulnerable to any pharmacological aggression likely to have a negative impact on their development. The issues surrounding the use of

such products in adolescents are not the same as in adults. This period is one of the most difficult in life for adolescents themselves, but also for parents, teachers and educators. It can be a very anxious time.Adolescent discomfort is caused by low self-esteem, provocative attitudes towards the family environment and repeated tests to prove one's worth. The search for models of identity that are different from those of the parents, the desire to escape family, social and school obligations, and the detachment f r o m   parental dependence encourage a stronger expression of physiological discomfort.

I-2-1-2- Gender

In our study, 96.6% of patients were male. Several studies [3, 29, 47-56] have shown that cannabis use is more common among men than women.Gender is one of the factors influencing illicit drug use. According to Eurobarometer [57], men are more likely to take drugs than women. Most men hope to forget their problems by using psychoactive substances. Gender is one of the risk factors for cannabis use.

I-2-1-3- Profession

Of our samples, 56.8% were farmers and farm workers.force. Farmers in Madagascar account for 80% of the working population [58]. According to a study carried out in Antsiranana by Randrianantenaina [6] on the epidemiological profile of illicit drug users admitted to the Morafeno psychiatric ward, 36.18% of drug users were farmers and forced labourers.According to the study by Rhandour in Morocco [56], and by Kazour et al in Lebanon [55], the majority of consumers have not had a job According to a study by Guillem et al [50], in France, 51.9% of consumers do not have a prescription.no work.In Madagascar, heavy labour is an unstable profession, and belongs mainly to people of low intellectual and socio-economic status. This work requires energy. Cannabis is often used for its euphoric, energising and anxiolytic properties.In our study, civil servants had a rate of 1.1%, which proves that commitment and responsibility are protective factors against cannabis use.

I-2-1-4-Marital status

In our study, 80.7% of cannabis-using patients were single.The study by Mabrouk et al [3] in Tunisia was almost equal to our study, with 81.6% of cannabis users being single.The results reported by other authors [49, 50, 55, 56] showed above all that single people used cannabis more often than married people.According to the study conducted by Elghazouani et al [33], the majority of addicts using psychoactive substances were single.Our results are similar to those in the literature. Single status is one of the risk factors for drug use, including cannabis. Single people feel free and very sensitive to the various festivities. Conversely, cannabis use can be the cause of celibacy. When the partner uses cannabis regularly, communication between the couple becomes heavy and complicated, as the partner's euphoric mood is transformed into a depressive one. In a state of dependence, all he or she cares about is immediate pleasure and runs away from any situation or context that takes him or her away from his or her primary goal: to have fun, to think of nothing and above all not to listen to his or her partner's criticism or advice.Physical violence is another aggravating factor in the relationship when one or both spouses use cannabis. On days when cannabis is used, the spouse is more exposed to physical violence than on sober days.

I-2-1-5-Level of study

In our study, 52.3% of cannabis users had secondary education and 35.2% had primary education.According to the study by Rhandour [56], the educational level of these patients is between primary and secondary school. According to a study by Radia [49], the majority of cannabis-using patients in Morocco (47%) were still at secondary school Another study by Alson [29] was similar to our study, with a rate of 58% having secondary education. The majority of cases indicated that the secondary level presented a risk. In our country's education system, the lesson on drug addiction is given in class 3eme . Yet most young cannabis addicts have already tried cannabis before reaching this class. What's more, low socio-economic status means that they drop out of school before the age of 3^e . The curriculum and quality of the school play a major role in the development of drug use problems and school drop-out. Dropping out of school is generally the result of a long process of disengagement on the part of a student who is dissatisfied with his or her school, the culmination of a gradual deterioration in the relationship between school and student: failures, absenteeism, vandalism, suspensions and expulsions.

I-2-1-6- Siblings

In our study, cadets were the most affected, with a rate of 54.5%. Younger children tend to get little attention from their parents. That's why they tend to surround themselves with lots of friends. The youngest child is the riskiest compared to the oldest and youngest. In our study, we had 15.9% younger children and 29% older children. This can be explained by the process of personality formation.The eldest child is often responsible for the other children in the family. It is up to them to set an example. As the youngest child is the youngest, he or she benefits from a certain parental laxity, as the parents trust each other more in their role [59]. Middle children tend to feel neglected by their parents. They are very sociable and know how to adapt to everyone. This adaptation attracts them to a group of delinquents in the belief that they do not always receive the attention that the eldest and youngest have received.

I-2-1-7-Background judiciaire

According to our study, we found that 93.2% of consumers had no forensic history and only 6.8% said they had a history with the law. On the contrary, according to a study by Oulmidi [60] on the epidemiological profile of psychoactive substance users attending the Marrakech addictology centre, 58% of users had a history of contact with the law, while 42% denied any contact with the authorities. According to a study by Randrianantenaina [6], 3.9% of drug users had a criminal record. Cannabis is not only one of the most widely used illicit psychoactive substances in the world, it is also one of the most widely used drugs in our city [6]. Our society is tolerant of the antisocial acts associated with cannabis use. This tolerance arises when there are arrangements with the victims and when the first crisis occurs. This is why the criminal record is weak and cases do not go to court.

I-2-2-Demographic characteristics of parents
I-2-2-1-Parenthood and marital status

In our study, the majority of patients' parents (63.6%) were single. Of these, 31.8% were raised by single mothers.According to Cascone's study in Argentina [61], 41% of adolescents had lived in a single-parent family, 33% had been brought up by single mothers, and that 67% of families have gone through a separation process, linked to divorce or placement.Inadequate parental education leads to psychological disorders, which in turn lead to poor adaptation to society. Parents play a vital role. Family composition is also reported to be an important factor in the development and use of psychoactive substances, particularly cannabis. A positive relationship and open communication between parents and young people are protective factors [62]. Adolescents from single-parent families show a significantly higher level of drug use than those living with both parents. Sometimes, the stress caused by difficult family relationships, conflicts or separations has an impact on cannabis use. Single-parent families, particularly single mothers, are unable to bring up their children on their own. This situation makes it easier for teenagers to become estranged from their family unit. Tired mothers who come home in the evening are unable to carry out their duties within the family. This underlines the importance of a father's role in a family, as protector and educator, to initiate and support children's self-control and to help them channel and control their aggression towards positive expression. According to the Shek study in the United States, the association between family functioning during childhood and social adjustment in adolescence has also been demonstrated, particularly with regard to behavioural problems. In a study of adolescents from disadvantaged backgrounds, family functioning (parental caregiving skills, presence of conflict within the family) was associated with the adolescent's psychological well-being, satisfaction with life, self-esteem and ability to adjust to school life [63].The family is a source of protective factors against psychological disorders in children and adolescents, as it forms the basis of the socialisation process.

I-2-2-2-Toxic habits

Our study revealed that 44.4% of consumers' parents had smoked. The study by Lochbuehler et al [64] and Ball et al [65] showed that having at least one parent who smokes and exposure to smoking at home constitute a social influence on cannabis.Drug use by parents poses a major risk to their children. Parents are role models for their children. Parents have a huge responsibility for shaping their children's lives. We believe that the family is the ideal place for educating children about the different kinds of drugs.

I-2-2-3- Profession

In our study, we found that 71.6% of consumers' parents were farmers and heavy labourers. Exhausted by their hard work during the day, these parents are no longer able to look after their children properly when they return home. What's more, most of the people doing this work are illiterate. But there are also those who stopped at primary school, and very few of those who have reached upper secondary school, if any, have not finished lower secondary school.

I-2-3-Group frequented and mode of consumption

In our study, all the users frequented other users. Of these, 93.2% smoked in groups.In France, the study by Bello et al [66] found that 83% of people consumed drugs in groups.The study by Karl and Regina [67] showed that almost all cannabis users had at least a few friends who used cannabis, whereas 55% of non-users reported having only one user among their friends. According to the study by Baumann and Enett [68], it is easier for adolescents to start using cannabis if at least one of their close friends is already using it. Cannabis consumption is part of socialising and festivities. This substance is used as a rite of passage to belong to a group. The more frequent the group, the higher the risk of using cannabis.

I-2-4-Training and awareness campaign on cannabis

According to our study, the majority of users (77.3%) have not had any education about cannabis and 22.7% have had some education during their studies. The majority of users in our study remained at secondary and primary level. In addition, the lack of family and social education and ignorance of the effects of cannabis increase the prevalence of users.

I-3-Data on cannabis

I-3-1- Age of onset of cannabis use

According to our study, the age of first exposure to cannabis was between 11 and 15 years, with a rate of 46.6%. According to the study by Akré et al [36] on cannabis use patterns among adolescents in France, the majority began using cannabis between the ages of 12 and 17. Some are not exactly sure of their age.

According to Randrianantenaina's study [6], 61.15% of users started taking drugs before the age of 18. This result is very high compared with that of Oumar in Mali, who found that 37.5% of users had started taking drugs under the age of 18 [69].This is often explained by the characteristics of vulnerability specific to this age group, as well as the environmental factors that accentuate this vulnerability. In the process of developing their identity, adolescents have to This is a time when they are rediscovering their environment and experimenting with different behaviours that provide stimulation and sensations, sometimes leading them to use psychoactive substances, including cannabis. This is the period when peers take on considerable importance as reassuring peers, and when the search for identifying markers is a priority. Being accepted into the peer group can be vital.

I-3-2-Mode of

Our study shows that 100% of users took cannabis by inhalation, all of them in the form of smoke.According to several studies, such as that by Grotenhermen [17], in Germany, the The respiratory route was the main route of administration. In all consumer countries, including our own, this route is easier to use than the other routes, because it is the most accessible and the least expensive. What's more, the other forms are rare and not available in our country.

I-3-3-Frequency of use and frequency of cannabis use for the regular users

According to our study, 95.5% of cannabis patients were regular users. Of the 84 patients who used cannabis regularly, 51.2% used it once a day. All the patients smoked one joint per dose.According to the study by Akré et al [36], 72.7% of users smoked several joints a day and 18.2% were occasional users. According to the study by Bello et al [66], in France, 78% of consumers smoked at least once a day.According to the study by Mabrouk et al [3], the majority of cannabis users in Tunisia were daily users. This result shows that most users consumed at least once a day. This can be explained by the fact that the cost is not high, and by the presence of dependence. What's more, the product is easily accessible. The more friends there are who use it, the easier it is to access. Dependence is due to an imbalance in neurobiological functioning following regular use. This imbalance leads to the desire to use the substance again, to avoid the unpleasant effects of stopping taking it.

I-3-4-Rationale for consumption

In our study, the predominant reason for consumption was group influence at a rate of 62.5%.According to the study by Poulin et al [70], 75% of cannabis use occurs in social situations such as group influence. The risk of use is higher when adolescents associate with peers who use cannabis.According to the Obradovic study [48], in France, 60% of patients who used cannabis were looking for pleasure and enjoyment.The reason for consumption also depends on the geographical and cultural context. The social and cultural influence of the group has also been identified as being factors associated with the onset of cannabis use [63]. It seems that these young people are tempted to take drugs by pressure from their friends, by curiosity or by imitating others, and by fear of being isolated from their group of friends. Influence by others has been identified as a cause of drug-taking by individuals. This influence can be fostered by low self-esteem and a need to feel recognised by those around them, by their friends and family.

I-3-5- Age of consumption

The average duration of use was 7.68 years, with a standard deviation of 4.35. The majority of users (64.8%) had been using cannabis for 1-10 years. According to the study by Guillem et al [50], after 12 months of cannabis use, 40% of users developed anxiety and mood disorders.According to the study by Potvin et al [71], after 15 years of use, users are at risk of developing schizophrenia. Our study falls somewhere between these two literatures. The majority of patients are unable to identify their first contact with cannabis. The psychoactive substances we consume act directly on the brain by modifying the behaviour, moods, perceptions and mental activity of users. Over the years, cannabis use leads to amotivational syndrome, manifested by widespread apathy, lack of attention, loss of productivity and lack of perseverance. Cannabis abuse increases the risk of chronicity and behavioural disorders involving criminal acts. Patients are often admitted to hospital only when they present more psychotic symptoms or behavioural disorders that make it difficult for them to integrate into society.

I-3-6- Associated substances

In our study, 44.3% of users associated cannabis with alcohol and tobacco. According to the study by Guillem et al [50] and Karila et al [72], tobacco was the most common substance used in the study.most frequently associated with cannabis.The results of other authors [3, 29, 49, 54, 56] showed that cannabis use was associated with alcohol and tobacco.Young people start their drug use trajectory with substances (tobacco and alcohol) before starting to use illegal substances,especially cannabis. We must always look for the possibility of multiple use among users of psychoactive substances, and raise awareness of the harmful psychological and somatic consequences of cannabis among tobacco and alcohol users. Consumption is often combined, either as a result of a training effect, or in search of a thrill, or to attenuate the effects of certain substances.

I-4- Clinical data

I-4-1-Distribution of patients by reason for admission

In our study, 80.7% were admitted for behavioural problems. This The result is almost identical to the Radia study.According to the study by Radia [49], the reason for admission was dominated by disorders of miscellaneous behaviour, with a rate of 80.6% of admissions.According to the study by Alson [26], the majority of admissions were for behavioural problems, with a rate of 85%.

Based on these results, it is necessary to request a biological sample in the event of a behavioural disorder to rule out the use of cannabis or other psychoactive substances as the first cause. Cannabis use must now be systematically investigated and assessed in the same way as tobacco or alcohol misuse or abuse of psychotropic drugs.

I-4-2-Distribution according to clinical manifestation

In our study, the majority were psychotic, accounting for 77.3% of our samples, and all were delusional. Polymorphic themes and ideas of grandeur were the most frequent, and 94.1% presented hallucinations, the most frequent of which were auditory and visual hallucinations, and 4.4% presented deficits.According to Radia's study [49], 94% of patients who used cannabis presented delusional syndromes, the most frequent theme of which was persecution. and multiple themes, and 41.7% presented with hallucinations, mainly auditory. Around 17% showed deficit signs.In Alson's study [26], 88.75% of the patients studied presented delusional syndromes, the most common themes of which were persecution and multiple themes. Approximately 94% of patients presented with hallucinations, the most frequent of which was auditory hallucination, and only 2.5% presented with deficit signs.Cannabis can be problematic and addictive, with harmful consequences for the individual. Heavy use leads to toxic psychosis. This is characterised by delusions, paranoia and hallucinations. The harmful consequences of such use are becoming more widespread, and healthcare professionals need to be aware of them in order to deal more effectively with these problems, first and foremost by spotting them early. When faced with an auditory or visual hallucination, toxicity tests should be requested for suspected drugs, including cannabis. The extremely significant changes in cannabis use and the damaging health and social consequences of this use require a rapid readjustment of society's perceptions.

I-4-3-Psychiatric history

In our study, 62.5% of users had no psychiatric history.In the study conducted by Guillem et al [50], 52% of cannabis-using patients had someone in their family with a psychiatric disorder. And 73% of cannabis-using patients had already had a psychiatric disorder in their lifetime.According to the study by Frascarelli et al [52], more than the majority of cannabis-using patients had a family history of psychiatric disorders.In Radia's study [49], only 11.1% of patients had a family history of psychiatric pathology and 73.3% had already had a psychiatric disorder in their lifetime.In the study by Mabrouk et al [3], 25.5% of consultants had a family history of psychiatric pathology and 28.8% had a personal history of psychiatric disorders.In Alson's study [26], 32% of patients had no personal or family history of family. Our results are better than those in the literature. Information on patients' families is not always complete. Secondly, in our department, patients' families cover all the costs of hospitalisation (accommodation, medication, food). The long duration of treatment and the cost of psychotropic drugs are a source of disruption to treatment, which means that patients' families are not motivated to go to the psychiatric department. Social representations of mental disorders and the stigma attached to patients suffering from mental disorders vary. Some people see them as manifestations of diabolical forces, evil spirits or possession. This is why some families and friends refuse to admit patients.

II- SUGGESTIONS

Cannabis use causes psychosis and creates problems for the family, society and the state. Cannabis use has evolved into mass consumption. Dependence is caused by an imbalance in neurobiological functioning following consumption. Ignorance of the dangers of cannabis use is a source of the spread of consumption throughout society. Faced with this situation, it would be necessary to take into account the following perspectives to better solve this problem.

On the research plan

- Increase sample data and study duration

- Extend the study to include different possible services and locations such as the home young.

- Completing clinical records correctly for all patients entering the department.

In practice

- Introduce THC testing as one of the check-ups to confirm the use of cannabis by patients presenting behavioural problems on admission to the department.
- Improving the care system :

✓ Strengthen the teams involved (doctors, psychologists, team leaders, health educators, moral values educators).
✓ Make psychotropic drugs more widely available and accessible to the general public.
✓ Inform the families of cannabis-using patients about the dangers of this substance at every consultation.
✓ A daily reminder of the Information Education Communication (IEC) against cannabis use in the department, together with psycho-education for patients and on-call staff.

On education

- Strengthening basic education :

✓ Advise all parents to send their children to school so that they can receive a basic education.
✓ Teachers and parents must set a good example by

abstaining from cannabis.

- Incorporate lessons on the harmful effects of cannabis use into the

general education programme from the end of primary school.

- Reinforce at every parents' meeting at school the need for dialogue between

parents and children talking about the dangers of drugs, including cannabis.

- Encourage students to continue their studies by giving bonuses to the best students in each class per school.

In social terms

- Training parents:

✓ Remind parents of the importance of the family.

✓ Create a parents' association against drug use.

✓ Set an example for the child by avoiding all psychoactive substances.

- Helping young people prepare for a future without cannabis and adopt better habits:
✓ Create associations and leisure centres to help teenagers from very disadvantaged families.
✓ Create leisure centres such as sports grounds, swimming pools, cultural centres, music and cinema.
✓ Organise competitions in the urban environment on the theme of "anti-cannabis" with the aim of reducing cannabis use in this environment.
✓ Creating jobs for unemployed young people.
✓ Building multi-disciplinary sports pitches in each neighbourhood, and organising competitive tournaments for all age groups.
- Improving the drug control system :

✓ Prohibit the planting and block the free movement of cannabis in Madagascar's Northern Region by mobilising the agents responsible.
✓ Introduce a highly effective control system both at airports and on the roads.
✓ Form teams with officers responsible for drug control (consumption, trafficking, cultivation).
✓ Strengthen measures for the effective application of the provisions of the law on drug use.
- Stepping up the cannabis education campaign:

✓ Train groups of educators to carry out Information Education Communication (IEC) activities against cannabis use at community level, within associations and religious entities.
✓ Create neighbourhood associations against cannabis use.

✓ Create cannabis detox centres in different districts if possible.
✓ Create a television or radio programme on the dangers of cannabis.

CONCLUSION

Cannabis is the most widely used illicit substance in the world. Its use poses a real public health problem. This leads us to examine the socio-familial factors associated with cannabis abuse and to assess the types of substances associated with cannabis.This study enabled us to describe the socio-familial factors that influence cannabis use. Cannabis is of interest to a number of individuals, including males, young people in groups, single people, people with low socio-economic and intellectual levels, and single parents, and its use is often associated with tobacco and alcohol.During the course of the study, we were faced with a number of obstacles, the most difficult of which was the lack of biological evidence to confirm cannabis use. In addition, the single-centre nature of the study meant that it did not reflect all the socio-familial factors of the general population of the city of Antsiranana.We feel it is necessary to put forward a few suggestions for combating this scourge. Firstly, through awareness and information campaigns, we need to make the general public aware that the problem exists. The best strategy for combating the use of cannabis is education. A number of players need to be mobilised, including parents, teachers, the community, religious bodies and associations, to put in place a strategy for early detection of at-risk or vulnerable populations. It is also necessary to set up a leisure centre within each company so that young people can enjoy themselves, and to create jobs adapted to the capacity of young people. An improved service and care system could facilitate cannabis withdrawal treatment.It is desirable to cooperate with laboratories to facilitate the availability of and the accessibility of THC dosing.

BIBLIOGRAPHICAL REFERENCES

1. Drugs and addictive behaviours. Inpes; editions, December 2014: 224 p.

2. World Health Organization. Cannabis: report on its effects on health and society. 2016. Available at www.who.int .

3. Mabrouk H, Mechria H, Merchia A, Douki W, Gaha L, Najjar MF. Cannabis use in a central Tunisian region. Sante 2011; 21: 233-9. DOI : 10.1684/san.2011.0274.

4. Gruber AJ, Pope HG. Marijuana use among adolescents. Pedatr Clin North Am 2002; 49:389-413.

5. Fergusson DM, Horwood LJ. Cannabis use and dependence in a New Zealand birth cohort. N Z Med J 2000; 113:156-8.

6. Randrianantenaina VC. Profil épidémiologique des usagers de drogues illicites admis au service de psychiatrie de Morafeno [Thesis]. Médecine Humaine : Antsiranana ; 2019. 45p.

7. Actualités santé publique France. Inpes. 2016. Available at https://www.santépubliquefrance.fr

8. Blecha L, Benyamina A. Cannabis and psychiatric disorders, L'information psychiatrique 2009; 85 :641-5. DOI:10.391/inpsy.8507.0641

9. Raobijaona H A. Jeunes et toxicomanie à Antananarivo. Antananarivo: Bulletin d'Information sur la population de Madagascar, 2007; 26: 1.

10. Republic of Madagascar. Control of narcotics, psychotropic substances and precursors in Madagascar. Antananarivo Official Journal of 04 November 1997

11. Gaulier JM. Cannabis: the biologist's new challenges. Revue Francophonie des laboratoires-February 2016; 479

12. Phan O, Corcos M, Girardon N, Nezelof S, Jeammet P. Cannabis abuse and dependence in adolescence. EMC-Psychiatrie; 2005; 2: 207-24

13. Constentin J. Neurobiology of cannabis. La lettre du psychiatre. March-April 2012; VII; 2

14. Goulle JP, Guerbet M. Key features of delta-9 tetrahydrocannabinol pharmacokinetics; new synthetic cannabinoids; cannabis and road safety. Bull.Acad.Natle.Méd.2014; 3 :541-57

15. Lauwagie S, Stern E, Millet R, Depreux P. Cannabinoids and cannabinoid receptor pharmacology. Lettre du pharmacologue.2006; 20; 3

16. Derkinderen P, Valijent E, Darcel F, Damier P, Girault JA. Cannabis and cannabinoid receptors: from physiology to therapeutic possibilities. Rev Neurol Paris ; 2004 ; 160 :6-7 : 639-49

17. Grotenhermen F. Cannabinoids and the endocannabinoid system. Cannabinoids. 2006; 1(1) :10-5

18. Inserm. Cannabis, what effects on behaviour and health. Expertise collective.2001; 117-42

19. Alvarez JL, Pape E, Stanislas GD, knapp. A. Synthetic cannabinoids:

pharmacological aspects.TOXAC 2014

20. Chadya A. Cannabis-induced psychotic disorders: a12-month longitudinal study[thesis]. Psychiatry: Morocco; 2012.96p

21. United Nations Office on Drugs and Crime. World Drug Report. 2015. Available at https://www.unodc.org/doc/wdr2015

22. United Nations Office on Drugs and Crime. World Drug Report. 2012. Available at https://www.unodc.org/doc/wdr2012

23. United Nations Office on Drugs and Crime. World Drug Report. 2016. Available at https://www.unodc.org/doc/wdr2016

24. United Nations Office on Drugs and Crime. World Drug Report. 2004. Available at https://www.unodc.org/doc/wdr2004

25. Beck F, Devraux A, Du Roscat E, Karine GM, Marie GB, Kern L, Krebs MO, et al. Addictive behaviour in adolescents-use, prevention and support. Editions Inserm, 2014 :25

26. European Monitoring Centre for Drugs and Drug Addiction. European report on drugs, trends and developments. 2107. Luxembourg. Publications Office of the European Union.

27. United Nations Office on Drugs and Crime. World Drug Report 2009. Available at https://www.unodc.org/doc/wdr2009

28. United Nations Office on Drugs and Crime. Cannabis in Africa. 2007. Available at https:// www.unodc.org/document/can_Afr_FR_09_11_07

29. Alson RE. Sociodemographic and clinical factors related to cannabis use [Thesis]. Médecine Humaine : Antananarivo ; 2018.53p

30. Ratobimanankasina L, Rajaonarison BH, Raharivelo A, Andriambao DS. Profil épidémiologique de la toxicomanie au lycée d'Antananarivo: à propos de 600 cas, first SOMAP National Congress, Rev.Med. Madag.2013; 3(2) :294-7.

31. Phan O, Obradovic I, Har A. Cannabis abuse and dependence in adolescence.Arch Pediatr. 2016

32. Thomas P , Amad A , Fovet .Schizophrenia and addiction: the links dangerous.L'encéphale 2016; 12: 3S18-3S22

33. Elghazouani F, Aarab C, Lohlou F, Elrhazi K, Aalouane R, Rammouz R. Substance use in patients hospitalized for schizophrenic relapse. Ann Méd Psychol. 2015

34. Kolliakou A, Joseph C, Ismail K, et al. Why do patients with psychosis use cannabis and are they ready to change their use? Int J Dev Neurosci 2011;29:335-46

35. Favrode J. Motivational interventions: psychosis and cannabis. Encéphale 2009; supplement 6 :S209-S213

36. Akré C, Michaud PA, Suris JC. Patterns of cannabis use among adolescents: a qualitative study. IUMSP (Lausanne, University Institute of Social and Preventive Medicine), Lausanne, 2008.

37. Grotenhermen F. Cannabis in medicine: a practical guide to the medical applications of cannabis and THC. Sélestat: Indica; 2009.

38. Michel G, Purper-Ouakil D, Mouren-Siméoni CM. Clinic and research on

conduites à risques chez l'adolescent. Elsevier; 2006; 54: 62-76

39. Michel G, Purper-Ouakil D, Mouren-Siméoni CM. Risk factors for psychoactive substance use in adolescence. Ann Méd Psychol. 2001; 159 :622-31
40. Karila L, Reynaud M. Traité d'addictologie.2ᵉ edition. Paris: Lavoisier Médecine science.2016
41. Laqueille X. The cannabis is a factor of vulnerability to schizophrenic disorders? Arch Pediatr. 2009; 16: 1302-05
42. Potvin S, Stip E, Roy JY. Schizophrenia and cannabinoids: clinical, experimental and biological data. Erudit; 2004; 2;2.DOI: 10.7202/008536ar
43. Dervaux A, Krebs MO, Laqueille X. Cognitive and psychiatric disorders associated with cannabis use. Bull.Acad. natle Méd, 2014 ; 198 ; 3 :559-77
44. Laqueille X, Launay C, Kanit M. Psychiatric and somatic disorders induced by cannabis. Ann Pharm Fr 2008; 66 :245-54
45. Benyamina A, Blecha L. The effects of cannabis on health. Ann Méd Psychol; 2009; 167: 514-17

46. Jouanjus. Identifying the serious complications associated with substance use psychoactive [thesis]. Pharmacology: Toulouse. 2013. 180p.
47. Geus CH, DE Longueville X, Schepens P. Psychotic disorder and cannabis use: a retrospective study. Louvain médical. 2004

48. Obradovic I. Consultation cannabis: enquête sur les personnes accueillies en 2005. Saint Denis: OFDT edition. 2006

49. Radia T. Psychotic disorder and cannabis use: about 60 cases [thesis]. Psychiatry. Rabat, Morocco.2008.196p

50. Guillem E, Pelissolo A, Vorspan F, Bouchez-Arbabzadeh S, Lépine JP. Sociodemographic factors, addictive behaviours and psychiatric comorbidity in cannabis users seen in specialist clinics. L'encéphale 2009 ;35 ; 226-33

51. Tessier S, M. sc. Cannabis use in Quebec and Canada: portrait and evolution. Inspq. 2017. Available at https://www.inspq.qc.ca
52. Frascarelli M, Quartini A, Tomassini L, Russo P, Zullo D, Manuali G et al. Cannabis use related to early psychotic onset: Role of premorbid function. Neuroscience letters 633; 2016; 55-61

53. Baraldi R, Jourbert K, Bordeleau M. To consume or not to consume cannabis: a look at the consumption profile of Quebecers. Zoom santé. 2016 ; 60. Institut de la statistique du Québec available at https://www.sta.gouv.qc.ca

54. Beck F, Legleye S, Spilka S. Cannabis - essential data: usage levels and profiles of users in France in 2005. Ofdt.2007 ;20-9

55. Kazour F, Awaida C, Souaiby L, Richa S. Research into the association between abuse and bipolarity : study of a sample of patients hospitalised with bipolar disorder. Encéphale. 2016

56. Rhandour T. Prevalence of cannabis use among schizophrenic patients

hospitalised at the Ibn Hassan Hospital in Fez. [Dissertation]. Public health epidemiology course. Morocco. 2014. 40p.

57. EOS Gallup Europe. Young people and drugs. Report. Flash EB. 2004 June ; 158 :1-77. Available at ec.europa.eu/public_opinion/flash/fl158_en.pdf

58. Ministry of Agriculture, Food and Forestry. Agricultural policies in around the world. Country sheet - Madagascar. 2015

59. Marika S. Your birth order influences your personality [online]. 2020 March [consulted on 09/06/2021] available at URL: http://www.salutbonjour.ca
60. Oulmidi A. Epidemiological profile of psychoactive substance users attending the Marrakech addictology centre [Thesis]. Psychiatry: Marrakech; 2016. 100p

61. Cascone P. Cannabis dependence in adolescents leaving school. [Thesis]. Psychology: Geneva; 2007. 243p
62. El Khoury M. Gestion de soi et addiction à la drogue : Approche analyticosystémique d'un groupe de jeunes drogués en situation thérapeutique (Thesis in Psychology - Clinical Psycholopathology). University of Strasbourg, Strasbourg, France. 2016
63. Shek D. The relation of Parental Qualities to psychological Well-Being, Alcohol Adjustment, and Problem Behavior in Chinese Adolescents with Economic Disadvantage. The American Journal of Family Therapy (2002); 30(3), 215-230.

64. Lochbuehler K, Schuck K, Otten R, Ringlever L, Hiemstra M. Parental smoking and smoking cognitions among youth: a systematic review of the literature. European addiction research (2016). 22(4), 215-232. doi: 10.1159/000446022
65. Ball J, Sim D, & Edwards R. Addressing ethnic disparities in adolescent smoking: is reducing exposure to smoking in the home a key? Nicotine & tobacco research (2019). 21(4), 430-438. doi: 10.1093/ntr/nty053
66. Bello PY, Plancke L, Cagni G, et al. Les usagers fréquents de cannabis, éléments descriptifs, France. 2004. Bull Epidemiol Hebd 2005 ;20 :89-91.
67. Karl B, Regina F. The influence of peer groups on drug use: psychotropic drugs. 2003. 9 : 195-202.
68. Baumann KE, Enett ST. Peer influence on adolescent drug use. American Psychologist, 1994. 1(49), 820-831

69. Oumar M. Consumption of narcotics in a university environment [Thesis]. Psychiatry: Mali; 2015. 47p
70. Poulin F, Kiesner J, Pedersen S, & Dishion TJ. A short-term longitudinal analysis of friendship selection on early adolescent substance use. Journal of Adolescence. (2011) ; 34(2), 249-256. doi: 10.1016/j.adolescence.2010.05.006
71. Potvin S, Stip E, Roy JY. Schizophrenia and cannabinoids: clinical and biological data. Drogues, santé et societé. 2004; 2(2). https://doi.org/10.7202/008536ar

72. Karila L, Petit A, Zamdini R, Coscas S, Lowenstein W, Reynaud M. Tobacco consumption and substance use disorder: what should we do? Press Med. 2013; 42: 795-805

APPENDICES

FACT SHEET

File number:
Date of admission :
Reason for admission: Clinical manifestations :
Patient's identity :
- Marital status :

Full name :

Age :

Gender :
- Occupation: Farmer/forced labourer☐student/ Pupil☐ Shopkeeper☐civil servant☐
- Marital status: Single☐As a couple☐

- Level of education: no schooling☐ primary☐secondary☐university☐
Personal history :

- Siblings :

- Judicial: yes☐ no☐

- Psychiatry: yes☐ no☐

- Parenthood: Father and mother☐father and stepmother☐mother and stepfather☐ grandparents☐ Other:

Family history :

Parents/ Guardian :		
-Marital status: Single☐	As a couple☐	
-Toxic habits: cannabis☐alcohol☐	tabac☐	cola☐
Others :		no☐

-Parents' occupation: Farmer/forced labourer☐

Retailer☐ Civil servant☐

Cannabis data :
➤ Consumption :

- Starting age :

- How to take: Inhalation: smoke☐ vaporisation☐

Oral route: pill☐ oil☐ Sublingual route: spray☐ Cutaneous route: cream☐

- Frequency: occasional☐regular (day/week/month) :

- Quantity :

- Reason: Group influence (pressure - farm performance - school performance) ☐

Pleasure seeking☐ Intolerance of frustration☐ Emotional shock☐ Aggression☐
- Age of consumption (year/month) :

➢ Smokes alone: yes☐ no☐

➢ Group attended: consumer☐non-consumer☐

➢ Cannabis education and awareness campaign: school☐ social☐
Family☐none☐
➢ Substances associated with cannabis: Alcohol☐ tobacco☐ khat☐ cola☐
Heroin☐ cocaine☐ other☐ none☐

VELIRANO

Eto anatrehan' Andriamanitra Andriananahary, eto anoloan'ireo mpampianatra ahy, sy ireo mpiara-mianatra tamiko eto amin'ity toeram-pianarana ity, ary eto anoloan'ny sarin i Hippocrate. Dia manome toky sy mianiana aho, fa hanaja lalandava ny fitsipika hitandrovana ny voninahitra sy ny fahamarinana eo ampanatontosana ny raharaham-pitsaboana.Hotsaboiko maimaimpoana ireo ory ary tsy hitaky saran'asa mihoatra noho ny rariny aho, tsy hiray tetika maizina na oviana na oviana ary na amin'iza na amin'iza aho mba hahazoana mizara ny karama mety ho azo.Raha tafiditra an-tranon'olona aho dia tsy hahita izay zavamiseho ao ny masoko, ka tanako ho ahy samy irery ny tsiambaratelo haboraka amiko ary ny asako tsy avelako hatao fitaovana hanatontosana zavatra mamoafady na hanamorana famitankeloka.Tsy ekeko ho efitra hanelanelana ny adidiko amin'ny olona tsaboiko ny antonjavatra ara-pinoana, ara-pirenena, arapirazanana, ara-pirehana ary ara-tsaranga.Hajaiko tanteraka ny ain'olombelona na dia vao notorontoronina aza, ary tsy hahazomampiasa ny fahalalako ho entimanohitra ny lalàn'ny maha olona aho na dia vozonana aza.Manaja sy mankasitraka ireo mpampianatra ahy aho, ka hampita amin'ny taranany ny fahaizana noraisiko tamin'izy ireo.Ho toavin'ny mpiara-belona amiko anie aho raha mahatanteraka ny velirano nataoko.Ho rakotry ny henatra sy ho rabirabian'ireo mpitsabo namako kosa aho raha mivadika amin'izany.

HIPPOCRATIC OATH

In the presence of the masters of this Faculty, of my fellow students, before the effigy of Hippocrates, I promise and swear in the name of the Supreme Being, to be faithful to the laws of honour and probity in the practice of Medicine. I will give my care free of charge to the needy and will never demand a fee above my work. I will not participate in any illegal fee-splitting. If I am admitted to the interior of a house, my eyes shall not see what goes on there, my tongue shall not speak of the secrets entrusted to me, and my status shall not be used to corrupt morals or encourage crime.I will not allow considerations of religion, nation, race, party or social class to come between my duty and my patient. I will maintain absolute respect for human life from the moment of conception. Even under threat, I will not allow my medical knowledge to be used against the laws of humanity.Respectful and grateful to my masters, I will give back to their children the instruction I received from their fathers.May men esteem me if I am faithful to my promises.That I will be shamed and despised by my colleagues if I fail to do so.

LICENCE TO PRINT

READ AND APPROVED

Thesis Director (Date, Signature, Stamp)

SEEN AND ALLOWED TO PRINT

The Dean of the Faculty of Medicine of Antsiranana
First and last name: BARIHELY Bienvenido

Title of thesis: " SOCIO-FAMILIAL FACTORS WHICH ARE TIED TO THE ABUSE OF CANNABIS CONSUMPTION SEEN IN MORAFENO PSYCHIATRY SERVICE "

Heading: PSYCHIATRY

Number of pages: 58

Number of tables: 10

Number of figures: 19

Number of appendices: 01Number de references bibliographical: 72

55

ABSTRACT

Justification: *Cannabis is the most consumed illicit substance in all around the word it seems that the young people is the most concerned about that.*
Target: *Describe the socio-familial factors correlate to the abuse of cannabis consume and evaluate the types of substances associated to the cannabis.*
Methods: *It's a retrospective study, descriptive and monocentric of cannabis consumer patients for 3 years. The treatment of data was done with Office Microsoft and Excel 2016 software.*
Results: *Among the 551 hospitalized patients, 137 have consumed cannabis, and 88 are selected. The average age was 24,43 years old and the majority of them are men (96,6%) that 93,2% have consumed with peer group. Their consumptions have interested the single- persons (80,7%), young people from single-parents family (63,6%) and the hard-workers (56,8%). The influence of group (62,5%) which dominates the causes of consumption. The substances associated the most frequent observed are alcohol and tobacco (44,3%).*
Conclusion: *Consumption of cannabis causes big problem of public health in Antsiranana, also in Madagascar. Knowing that factors linked to this consumption can brake its progress.*
Key words: *Cannabis, masculine gender, young, single, single-parent family, influence of group.*
Thesis director *: Professor RAHARIVELO Adeline*

Thesis reporter: *Doctor ZANADAORY*
Author's address : *Lot 255 MLE Lazaret Sud Antsiranana*

Full name: BARIHELY Bienvenido

Title of thesis: "SOCIO-FAMILY FACTORS RELATED TO DRUG ABUSE".

CANNABIS SEEN IN THE PSYCHIATRIC DEPARTMENT OF MORAFENO ANTSIRANANA "

Category : PSYCHIATRY

Number of pages: 58

Number of tables: 10

Number of figures: 19

Number of appendices: 01 Number of bibliographical references: 72

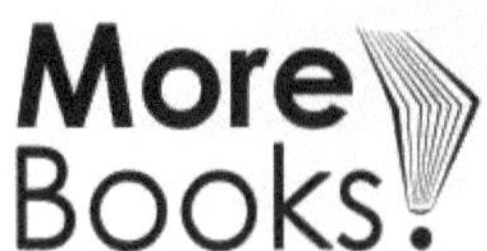

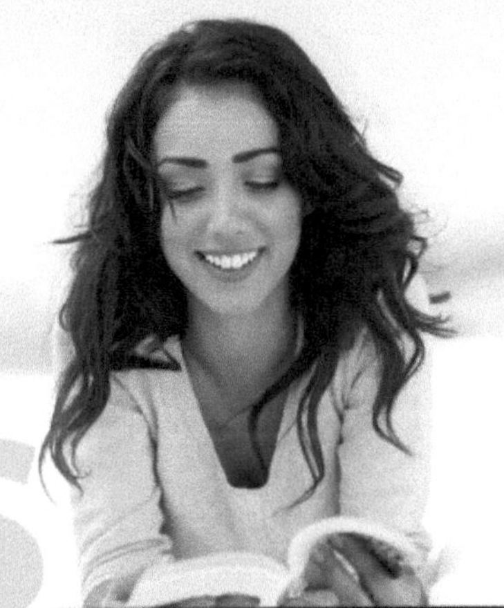

I want morebooks!

Buy your books fast and straightforward online - at one of world's fastest growing online book stores! Environmentally sound due to Print-on-Demand technologies.

Buy your books online at
www.morebooks.shop

Kaufen Sie Ihre Bücher schnell und unkompliziert online – auf einer der am schnellsten wachsenden Buchhandelsplattformen weltweit! Dank Print-On-Demand umwelt- und ressourcenschonend produziert.

Bücher schneller online kaufen
www.morebooks.shop

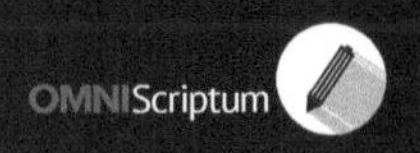

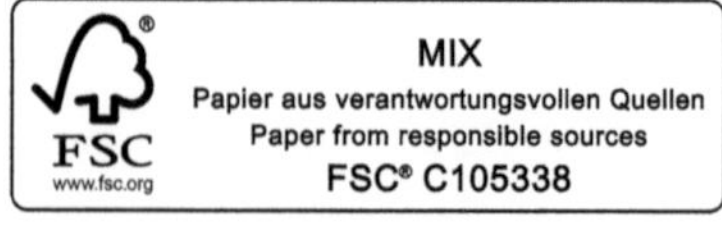

Printed by Books on Demand GmbH, Norderstedt / Germany